Nail Fungus Treatment

How to naturally cure nail fungus in 30 days

By: Adam Cooper

Copyright © 2016 Adam Cooper

All rights reserved.

This book is or any part of it may not be reproduced in any written, electronic, recording, or photocopying without written permission of the publisher or author having intellectual rights over the content of the book. The exception would be in the case of brief quotations embodied in the critical articles or reviews and pages where permission is specifically granted by the publisher or author.

Although every precaution has been taken to verify the accuracy of the information contained herein, the author and publisher assume no responsibility for any errors or omissions. No liability is assumed for any damage or damages that may result from the use of information contained herein.

Information contains in this book in solely for information purposes and does not intend in any way to replace professional medical and health advices rendered by practitioners in the field of medicine and you are further recommended to seek professional advice before using this material.

ISBN-10: 1539416097
ISBN-13: 978-1539416098

CONTENTS

1	You can cure nail fungus naturally	1
2	What is nail fungus	4
3	Don't ignore it!	9
4	What doctors recommend you to use	18
5	Cure nail fungus naturally	26
6	Get rid of nail fungus in 30 days	40
7	Prevent nail fungus from coming back	66
8	Conclusion	71

YOU CAN CURE NAIL FUNGUS NATURALLY

Nail fungus is an embarrassing condition that effects a large part of the adult population. The offensive odor and sight from nail fungus leaves many individuals hiding their feet constantly by never exposing them to the sun! Wearing closed toe shoes all ear round and dreading any social events that calls for exposed toes, such as the beach.

Hiding your feet isn't a solution and in fact can make the condition worse. What doesn't help is the fact that conventional western medicine can takes several months to rid this unsightly stubborn condition, with a high possibility of it reoccurring soon after. This is because most western medicine treatments don't address the root cause of nail fungus and instead seeks to rid the fungi on the surface of the nail itself. This method of treatment is superficial to say the least and is exactly the reason why most treatment methods take so long for results to appear and for the fungi to reappear.

This book will provide you a comprehensive outline of all the possible methods you can try to help yourself get rid of nail fungus once and for all. It will include the conventional western medicine treatments as well as a wealth of natural remedies that have been proven to improve and cure nail fungus.

The best possible solution to beating nail fungus is to understand it, and so this book will walk you through identifying nail fungus, treating nail fungus and preventing nail fungus.

The 30 day treatment outlined in this book aims to:

- Curb habits that encouraging nail fungus growth.
- Provide new habits that help prevent nail fungus to reoccur.

NAIL FUNGUS

- A detailed outline of actions to take for 30 days to cure or improve your condition.

WHAT IS NAIL FUNGUS

The Fungal infection, which is also known as "*tinea unguium* or *onychomycosis*" is a common disease that affects the finger and toenails.

This is manifested by discoloration, crumbling edges, and thickening of the nails, because the infection develops over time, the effects are not easily identified or associated to the nail fungi growing. The disease accounts for about 50% of nail abnormalities and around 6-8 percent of the adult population suffers from it in the United States alone.

Fungi are present everywhere in our surroundings, hence it is not unusual that some fungi and their spores are stuck on the surface of skin or inhaled and stored in the lungs. Fungi can grow rapidly, where there is moisture and warmth, when coupled with injury or skin irritations.

What Causes Nail Fungus Infections to Occur?

Most often, a group of fungi known as *dermatophytes* like *Candida Albicans* normally inhabits the intestines and is responsible for the occurrence of the nail fungal infection. Sometimes, yeasts and molds can also bring about this infection, and because a fungus doesn't necessarily need sunlight to survive, they can affect anyone exposed to it.

Pathogens, which cause nail fungus infection, can enter through your skin via tiny cuts and small spaces in between the nail and the nail bed. The fungus is grows easily when the nail serves a suitable moist and warm environment. Such as wearing shoes on a hot day or leaving feet damp after a shower.

The fungus can naturally overpopulate and bring

about athlete's foot, ringworm, and jock itch. Fungi can be spread to you, if you have been in contact with people who have fungi or even surfaces that have the fungi on it. Under the right conditions, fungi will affect your toenails more you're your fingernails because our shoes provide them with the perfect environment to grow and populate.

The infection may also be a result of having contact with an infected surface including garments, bed sheets, or towels. It can easily spread to other parts of the body by way of scratching, rubbing, and touching.

Tinea unguium infection has been associated with the use of *methacrylate,* which is used in attaching acrylic fingernails. So be careful when you have your nails manicured and pedicured. Tools that are not sanitized can aid in the transfer of fungi from one person to another, and this fungi will rapidly grow and infect your nails if given the right conditions to do so.

Types of Onychomycosis

Based on the origin of an infection within the nails, the organism that causes the infection on the surface of the nail, Onychomycosis is classified into the following types:

Distal or Lateral Subungual Onychomycosis
This is the most common form of O*nychomycosis*. It appears to be yellowish, whitish or brownish in color and usually starts under the edge or sides of the nail before it spreads over the entire nail. Though all nails are susceptible to it, the big toenail attracts it the most.

Proximal Subungual Onychomycosis
This type of infection affects the proximal nail fold and spreads distally.

Superficial Onychomycosis:
The fungus can invade the superficial layers of the nail and can go deeper into the nail plate. Lesions appear to be whitish and usually caused by *T. menta grophytes.*

Endonyx Onychomycosis

The nail bed is not involved in this type of infection. However, the infection can affect the interior portion of the nail plate. It the nail will appear darker, this type of infection is harder to treat with western medicine.

Totally Dystrophic Onychomycosis

The nail bed in this type of infection is thickened and raised with an evident amount of crumbling around the edge of the nail.

Yeast Onychomycosis

This may be a sign of underlying immunodeficiency. It is often caused by Candida and mostly affects fingernails than toenails.

Fungal Melanonychia

This is an uncommon type of infection, which causes brownish or blackish discoloration in the nail plate. This infection is brought about by melanin-producing molds including *Scytalidium*, *Exophiala*, and *Scytalidium*.

DON'T IGNORE IT

Are you aware that nail fungus infection is more common in women than in men? Our elderly people are more prone to this disease than younger individuals.

What are the Common Symptoms?

You can easily identify nails that are infected with the fungus as they appear thick, brittle, ragged, crumbled and a coloring that is yellowish or darker than natural. In worse cases, nail fungal infection can be painful, may emit a foul odor, and some people can experience *Onycholysis* or a condition that causes the nail to be separated from the nail bed.

Other symptoms may also include rashes or feeling of itchiness in a certain area of the body which is not affected by the fungus as it is more of an allergic reaction. These fungus-free lesions are known as *dermatophytids*.

Tinea infections usually appear like a red and scaly circular-shaped patch on the skin that is itchy and can spread easily. Hairs on the infected area often fall off as the skin cracks, leaving it prone to develop a secondary bacterial infection.

It's important to learn how to identify nail fungus during its early stages, as this is the best time to start treatment. Prolonging treatment gives the fungus a chance to deeply root itself to your nail, making treatment harder to get rid of it.

Here are some risk factors accounting for an increase possibility of nail fungal infection.

- Age - If you are over 65 years old
- Slow growth of nails
- Poor blood circulation
- Weak immune system
- Genetic disorder
- Heavy perspiration
- Walking barefoot in humid public places like pools, shower rooms, and gyms
- Injured or previously infected skin or nail
- Socks that prevent ventilation
- A workplace without proper ventilation resulting to heavy perspiration and an environment that is moist.
- Wearing of tight shoes causing your toes too close together
- Medical condition including AIDS, diabetes, circulation problem, etc.

which can weaken the immune system.

- Exercises that can lead to a repetitive minor cause of trauma to the hyponychium or that part where the finger tip attaches to the nail.

It is said that fungal infections are more rampant and severe in people taking antibiotics, contraceptives, corticosteroids, and immunosuppressant drugs. It has produced the same effects to those with immune diseases, endocrine disorders, and other medical conditions like obesity, diabetes mellitus, AIDS, leukemia, and major burns.

This is because most of the above listed medication weakens your body's natural ability to curb the nail infection's growth.

3 Growth Stages of Fungus Infection

Early Stage

It's difficult to detect a fungal infection while it's

still at the early stage as an infected person will not feel any discomfort or pain either in his hands or feet. However, you may be able to spot visible signs of fungus growth if you pay close attention. When detected early, it can help in the person's swift recovery from the infection by taking early action. Early signs can include discoloring of the finger or toenails. White or yellowish spots are evident on the edge of the nail or you can see some yellow streaks across it.

Many individuals fall into a trap of simply ignoring the situation at this early stage, thinking it will go away by itself or that the lack of discomfort means there's nothing to address. Don't fall into this trap. Early signs of infection means fungus has already embed itself to the nail and is actively growing.

Intermediate Stage

At this stage, the infected individual starts to feel some form of discomfort as the fungus can thoroughly cause a change in the coloring of the nail. The discoloring is more obvious and easily noticeable at this point. The nail also starts to change in shape, thickens and starts to show signs that it is separating from the nail bed. The edges will appear crusty, dry and disfigured.

Most people only start to worry at this stage as the visible symptoms of nail fungus starts to cause a real physical discomfort, nails that are starting to dislodge themselves away from the nail bed will become sore and tender to the touch. This makes putting on a sock, or wearing shoes uncomfortable.

This stage is also when the nail fungus starts to cause social problems by lowered confidence and or discomfort in social situations due to the visibility of the nail fungus.

The Advanced Stage

This is the stage when the nail had eventually separates itself from the nail bed entirely. The nail crumbles as the fungus has completely invaded it. The separation of the nail often results in exposed flesh underneath, which can cause an offensive odor to emit from the nail. This is a sign of a secondary infection occurring.

At this point, those suffering from the infection need to be aware of the problem and see a doctor as soon as possible while there are still some treatments options possible. The entire toe area needs to be treated first for the possibility of a new healthy nail to grow back. This book will not be able to address the advanced stages of nail fungus, only strong anti-fungul medicine can address your infection at this stage.

How Do I Know If I Have a Fungal Nail Infection?

Because there are some other infections that can imitate the symptoms of a nail fungus infection, the sure way to confirm that you have this disease is to check with your physician.

To be able to diagnose nail fungus, the doctor may examine some debris scraped from the underside of your nail. Diagnosis of a nail fungus infection can be made through a visual inspection.

Microscopy

Potassium Hydroxide (KOH) Stain is commonly used to detect the presence of the infection as it is inexpensive and easy to perform. Some samples of nail clippings or scrapings are dropped in the KOH solution and examined with the use of a microscope for the presence of the fungus.

Culture

This test is conducted to identify the exact type of nail fungus infection. By using fungal culture on *sabourad's* medium or *dermatophyte* test medium (SDTM). The fungus is allowed to grow and then be examined for identification.

The KOH test can quickly provide a result while the fungal culture can take several weeks before results are given back to you.

Physicians are also very careful with the examination because of a number of other medical conditions that can result in similar symptoms such as:

- Lichen Planus
- Psoriasis
- Contact Dermatitis
- Nail Bed Tumor
- Trauma
- Eczema
- Yellow Nail Syndrome

If your symptoms do not improve after 30 days following this book, please seek a physicians' medical advice as you may not have nail fungus, but instead another underlying medical condition.

WHAT DOCTORS RECOMMEND YOU TO USE

There are several medications available that will treat a light fungus nail infection if you spot it at its onset stage when the nail at this point is still not full exposed to the fungus.

As the fungus infection grows deeper into the nail, it will become more evident that the fungus has managed to set in. Your doctor may prescribe a stronger medication in such a case. This is normally the last stages of the intermediate stage of nail fungus.

One general rule of nail infection is this: The deeper the fungus has set in, the harder it is to get rid of. Therefore the number one rule to fighting nail fungus is treating is early.

Now, here are some of the most common prescription drugs that your doctor is likely to give you depending on the severity and type of infection.

Oral Medication

Oral antifungal medication work by encouraging the body to produce a new nail to replace the infected area. It also works to suppress the fungal growth simultaneously, which means the pace at which the infection grows is slower than the body's ability to remove and replace the nail.

Terbinafine

This drug is usually taken for a maximum of 12 weeks with one pill a day. In addition, the doctor may recommend "pulse dosing". This means you are to take the medicine every day for one week in a calendar month but not for the rest of the month. In pulse dosing, it could take up to 4 months before you can see any results.

Griseofulvin

This drug is taken twice per day until the nail infection is fully treated. For a more severe cases of infection, it is normal for the medicine to be taken for up to 18 months to eliminate the disease and prevent reoccurrence of the infection.

Fluconazole, Itraconazole, and Ketoconazole

These three drugs work in the same manner but can vary in reactions to different people. Therefore, follow only the doctor's prescription as he knows best. You can take this up to 18 months and may also use any of them with pulse dosing.

The above oral medication for nail fungus can be an expensive option due to the length of treatment required. The long treatment times required is due to doctors needing to balance the dosage to not bring about negative side effects, as these drugs are anti-fungal drugs that also suppresses your bodies ability to fight off other bacteria. Always follow your doctor's prescribed dosage as larger does will bring about negative side effects and lower doses will not kill of the fungus infection.

Topical Medication

Most topical agents will have a similar if not longer

treatment length as oral medication, however the method in which they work are starkly different. Topical treatments work to kill the fungus directly on the area instead of oral medication, which aims to replace the infected area with new healthy nail material.

Topical treatments are commonly not as strong and therefore not as effective compared to oral medication, but many people opt to try topical treatments first as they instinctively think direct application on the infected area will be the most effective. This is actually wrong and may waste valuable time in preventing your nail fungus infection from spreading further.

Over-the-counter antifungal creams are sold at most stores, you can also fine over the counter aerosol sprays. These type of medication can easily kill the fungus that causes the infection, however, since the fungus roots is buried deeper down into the inner skin, the medication can't get into the root, leaving the affected area untreated.

In short, this type of medication can control the symptoms but not the fungi itself. You will find your condition to appear as if it is improving to only find the fungus to constantly grow back once you stop treatment.

Laser Treatment

This treatment involves the use of a laser beam to penetrate the nails and kill the pathogens buried deep under the nail bed, which is causing the infection. The laser beam is supposed to pass through the nail without causing any damage to the skin or the surrounding area.

The new technology, like other treatment options, carries significant drawbacks that must be considered before opting for it.

Clinical trials aimed at the laser treatment effectiveness were done on a limited scale. The cost of the treatment is expensive and there is no guarantee for non-recurrence. There are some cases when a patient is required 3-4 visits and this entails a much higher cost. Lastly, because this technology is still on its onset stage, there is not much to prove that this technology will work for everybody.

However, laser treatment maybe the fastest and most convenient way to solve this embarrassing condition.

Debridement

This kind of treatment for nail fungus infection involves the nonsurgical removal of the infected area through a painless procedure. This treatment removes only the damaged or diseased nail and not any of the healthy part. However in some cases, your physician may decide the removal of the entire nail is required to ensure the fungus will not reappear again in the new nail that grows back.

To do this, the physician will first cover the normal skin around the infected nail with a piece of adhesive tape, which is of clothing material. A urea ointment is then applied directly on the surface of the nail before covering it with plastic and tape. The ointment is expected to soften the nail within 7-10 days. Be sure to keep the dressing dry during this period.

When the nail softens, the doctor will then remove the nail by lifting it apart from the nail bed or by cutting only the diseased portion of the nail.

Surgery

In severe infections, nails are required to be removed through surgery. The permanent removal of the infected nail will give way to treating the root of the fungus causing the infection and prevents the reoccurrence of the deformed nail.

In a surgical removal, the physician will loosening the skin around the nail fold to separate the nail from the nail bed or skin by inserting a tool under the nail. If only a part of the nail is affected, only that portion is cut and removed.

To avoid future recurrences of the nail fungus infection, the doctor can prevent the nail from growing back by destroying the nail matrix. To accomplish this, the doctor will be applying a chemical substance to the nail area after removing the infected nail plate. An antibiotic ointment is then applied to the wound and covered with gauze and adhesive plaster to cover the wound and avoid further infection.

For a few weeks after the surgery, dress your wound

regularly and apply antibiotic ointment. The wound should heal within a few weeks. A new nail will take 6-9 months to grow back.

A surgical removal is usually performed only when a large portion of the nail is diseased or damaged and when it causes you severe pain. In other cases, only the affected portion is removed and not the whole nail.

After the removal procedure, antifungal cream is applied to the remaining portion of the nail or oral antifungal medicine is prescribed.

CURE NAIL FUNGUS NATURALLY

30 Natural Home Remedy for Nail Fungus Infection

No one is able to ignore a nail fungal infection for too long and nobody would want to spend up to 18 months worth of medical bills for the medication to kill this fungal infection. They need a treatment that can work deeply into the nail to kill the fungus at its root.

Here are 30 natural home remedies for nail fungus infection which you can use daily for 30 days to effectively cure your nail fungus infection. Because of their natural elements, you can avoid side effects which are sometimes present in potent antifungal medications.

#1 - Apple Cider Vinegar

Take some water and mix it with equal amounts of apple cider vinegar. Soak the infected nail in the mixture for about half an hour on a regular basis. You can do this soak daily or as many times as required.

You can also make your own antifungal exfoliating scrub by adding some apple cider vinegar to just a small amount of ground rice flour. Mix the two ingredients to form a sticky mixture and apply some on the affected area while scrubbing gently. After a few minutes, wash with water.

#2 - Baking Soda

You will need:

- ½ cup of Epsom salt
- 4 cups of water
- ½ cup of white vinegar
- ¼ cup of hydrogen peroxide
- ½ cup of baking soda

Soak your infected nail in it for about 10 minutes. Wash your hands afterward and let it dry. Do this twice a day for several weeks to get rid of the infection.

As an alternative, prepare a pasty solution by mixing water and baking soda in a ratio of 1:2. Use the paste on the infected area using a cotton ball and leave it for 15 minutes before rinsing it off. Repeat the process two times in a day for about 2 weeks to see signs of improvement.

#3 - Listerine Mouthwash

Listerine mouthwash is not only effective in killing germs and bacteria in the mouth but also in your toenails. There are several compound substances present in Listerine including alcohol which serves as a strong antiseptic and keeps harmful fungi and bacteria away.

Take a small basin and fill it with an equal proportion of white vinegar and Listerine. Soak your toenail in it for approximately half an hour while scrubbing it gently. Rinse and repeat the same process 1-2 times in a day to keep the bacteria at bay. Just don't forget to thoroughly dry your toes especially the spaces in between the toes as moist and damp places are a good dwelling place for fungi.

#4 - Coconut Oil

Lauric acid and medium chain *triglycerides* are two ingredients present in the coconut oil which help break the cell wall of the fungus. Apply this mixture to the affected area to prevent fungus growth is very effective.

You can also choose to apply coconut oil onto your infected nail before choosing to soak your nail in one of the soaks listed in this book. This method can be helpful for individuals with thickened nails.

#5 - Garlic

Eating 1 or 2 cloves of crushed garlic a day will help treat your fungal infection. You can also mix it in equal proportion of garlic oil and vinegar and apply it on the toenail and then cover it with a bandage. Leave the bandage on for an hour before rinsing the solution off and drying the area clean. You can repeat this daily for as long as required.

Garlic is a natural anti-bacterial and anti-fungal that helps slows down fungal growth as well as prevent it.

#6 - Vitamin E

Apply Vitamin E Oil on the affected area especially under the nail. Apply daily for a quick recovery. Vitamin E is great for skin, hair and nails as it encourages the body to produce new cells.

#7 - Lemon Juice

Get a fresh lemon and extract the juice. Put some of the juice directly on the infected part for about 30 minutes before rinsing with warm water. Repeat it for a couple of times more to prevent the fungus from spreading. The acidity of lemon juice help kills the infection and soften the nail for other natural remedies to work more effectively.

#8 - White Vinegar

Combine white vinegar and lukewarm water in a ration of 1:2. Soak the infected fingers or toes in the prepared solution for 15 minutes. Rinse and let dry. Repeat the process 2 times daily to for skin pH restoration of the skin.

#9 - Vicks Vaporub

Using warm water, wash your feet and pat it dry. Apply *Vicks vaporub* on your infected toenails. Cover them with a bandage before wearing a sock to secure them. Do this twice a day for about 6-10 weeks until you see some improvements.

#10 - Turmeric

Make a paste by mixing turmeric and water. Spread this on the affected part and leave for a few minutes until dry. After a while, wash it with plain water.

In addition, prepare a diluted solution with turmeric oil and water in a ration of 1:3. Apply the solution on the infected nail and repeat the process to speed up the healing.

#11 - Onion

Slice an onion and rub it on the infected toes for several minutes. This is considered an effective natural remedy for fungus infection. Onions are naturally anti-septic which helps kills off the fungus on your nail.

#12 - Probiotic Foods

Increase your consumption of probiotic foods to get rid of nail fungus infection. Yogurt and Kefir can provide you the needed probiotics. However, by adding sugar or some artificial filler, you can somehow nourish the fungus. Avoid sweetened yogurt.

#13 - Tea Tree Oil

A few drops of the tea tree oil mixed with one teaspoon of coconut or olive oil when applied to the infected area can cure nail fungus infection. Let the solution seep into your skin and leave it there for about 10 minutes while gently scrubbing your toenails using a clean toothbrush. Repeat this process for 2-3 times a day.

#14 - Sodium Borate

This compound solution is commonly known as borax. Mix baking soda and sodium borate in equal proportion and dilute it with a small amount of water, enough to make a paste. Keep this aside while you wash your feet clean. Then spread the solution over the infected toenails, gently massaging it around the affected area. Try performing this house remedy 2-3 times a day for about 2 weeks.

#15 - Hydrogen Peroxide

One of the most common natural home remedies for foot fungus is Hydrogen peroxide. Mix water with the hydrogen Peroxide. A stronger preparation may cause some skin reactions and side effects so use a 3% solution and then dip your toes in it for around 2 minutes.

Other approaches include wiping the peroxide over the infected part for several times in a day. You may also spray it over the affected parts and allow it to go dry. Using this treatment is also effective for athlete's foot. This will help remove the fungus and one of the inexpensive treatments one can use.

#16 - Rubbing Alcohol

Rubbing alcohol which is often use as antiseptic has antifungal properties. Soak your feet in the solution for about 20 minutes to remove the fungus on your toenails.

Isopropyl alcohol can best beat fungus when applied to the area where the nail and the skin meet or under the nail so it can reach the nail bed. If you do this twice a day, after a few weeks you can see that the nail will be able to revert back to its normal color. However, along with alcohol, you must use other stronger antifungal like hydrogen peroxide to keep fungus from coming back.

Note that rubbing alcohol will also dry out the surrounding area.

#17 - Cornmeal

Place whole ground corn meal in a basin, about an inch deep then add 10 cups of water on it. Avoid mixing and just let it sit for about an hour. Then soak your feet in the mixture for 30 minutes to an hour. Do this two times a day.

#18 - Lemongrass Oil

Lemongrass has antifungal antibacterial properties. You can use the lemongrass oil to protect your toenails from further fungal infection while reducing the symptoms including distortion of nails, fragility, and the crumbling of nails. This is an effective remedy and you can apply this through any of the following ways.

- Add 12 drops of lemongrass oil to one ounce of grapeseed or coconut oil and apply it over infected areas.
- Drink a cup of lemongrass tea three times a day to heal the infection from the inside.

- For faster effect, compress the teabag on the infected part to clear it from fungus.

#19 - Oregano Oil

The oregano plant carries antifungal properties that can heal nail fungus infection. Add a few drops of oregano oil in 1 tsp of olive oil. Apply this mixture over the infected nail, seeing to it that it runs through the underside of the nail to seep through the nail bed. Leave it for about 30 minutes. After a few minutes, rinse it off. Repeat this remedy 2 times a day for 3 weeks.

Oil of Oregano is almost a well-rounded natural treatment by itself – it is antiseptic, antiviral, antibacterial, anti-parasitic, analgesic, and antifungal.

#20 - Lavender Oil

Make a mixture of 5 drops lavender oil and 5 drops of tea tree oil. Then apply this solution to the affected area using a cotton ball. Let it stay for about 10 minutes before rinsing it off. Repeat 1-3 times in a day to get rid of the fungi and prevent irritation.

#21 - Saltwater

Prepare some salted warm water in a basin and add hydrogen peroxide and then dip your feet in it. Stay there for around 30 minutes. Afterward, pat your feet dry and apply one or two drops of vinegar to your toenails. To heal the infection completely, repeat this process several times. This will destroy the fungus causing the infection.

#22 - Manuka Oil

Manuka oil is known as the best treatment for nail fungus infection. With just a few drops of this herbal oil, apply it directly to your infected nail. After applying the remedy, make sure that you cover your feet with cotton socks or any piece of fabric or gauze and leave it for an hour.

Another procedure of applying the treatment using *Manuka oil* is to take two quarts of lukewarm water and mix it with about 10 drops of *Manuka oil*. Then soak your feet in this solution for approximately 15 minutes to prevent further outgrowth of the fungus.

#23 -Black Walnut Salve

You can prepare the mixture by adding 8 drops of

tea tree oil, 1 cup of hydrogen peroxide, 1 box of sea salt, and black walnut hull. Mix all ingredients properly and soak the infected part in this solution for about 30 minutes. This will improve the condition of the infected nail.

#24 - Indian Lilac Oil

The antifungal properties of this substance moisturize and nourish the infected area while getting rid of the infection. Apply and massage the oil over the nail for treatment.

#25 - Olive Oil

Mix an equal proportion of olive oil and lemon juice and blend them well. Apply by massaging it over the infected area and wash off after a few hours. This remedy is sure to control the spread of infection on other parts.

#26 - Licorice

In a cup of boiled water, add 6 teaspoons of the powdered licorice. Leave the solution to a simmer over medium heat. After a few minutes, take it off the heat and let it pass through a strainer before applying the solution to your nails with the use of a cotton ball. Repeat this treatment three times every day for a fast recovery.

#27 - Castor Oil

For an effective treatment, simply soak a piece of cotton cloth in castor oil and wrap it around the infected nail or around your foot all night.

#28 - Pau D' Arco Tea

Use about 1-2 teaspoon of this herb and boil it in 1 cup of water for at least twenty minutes. Allow it to cool down and then soak your foot on it to get rid of the toenail fungus.

#29 - Iodine Tincture

Iodine Tincture may be one of the best home remedies we have for nail fungal infection. To strengthen the weakened nail that is affected by the infection, you can apply iodine tincture directly over it. However, before applying, wash the affected hands or feet with the infected nail and have it dried thoroughly.

Be sure to put the solution on top, underside, and underneath the nail. It is best applied before going to bed at night. Repeat this process for a week daily. Take note, however, that you must not use hydrogen peroxide on the nail that has been treated with iodine tincture.

#30 - Orange Oil

For treatment, you can apply orange oil on the infected area using a dropper. Let it stay for half an hour. Do this process 2-3 times a day for 2-3 months. Note that this solution may cause some reaction on some people; hence try it on a small portion of your skin before applying this remedy.

GET RID OF NAIL FUNGUS IN 30 DAYS

While there are many who are suffering from the inconvenience and suffering brought about by nail fungus infection, here's a natural way to get rid of nail fungus in 30 days.

As we have noted in the previous chapters; it is the *Candida Albicans* fungus that is responsible for nail fungus infection, it is, therefore, essential to integrate into our fungus treatment plan the characteristics of the Candida Albicans fungus.

The Candida Treatment involves 3 Major Elements

- The Cleansing Diet
- Probiotic Foods

- The Antifungals

The Cleansing Diet

An essential element in the Candida Treatment is the planning of your diet. The Candida diet plan involves switching to a low-sugar diet which can deprive the fungi of the food they need to grow and spread in your body. It also begins with a cleansing process to clear out Candida toxins. As the diet progresses and improvements are evident; you can gradually go back to foods like starchy vegetables and legumes.

Because sugar is the major cause of the *Candida Albicans*, the fungus responsible for the nail infection. Sugar is capable of starting the growing process of this fungus on our bodies, and this is the reason why it is the first element to be considered in the *Candida Treatment*. The fungus needs sugar to thrive and build their cell walls, expand their colonies, and transform into a more potent fungal form.

It is proven that carbohydrates are indispensable resources for fungi for their cellular growth and transformation from the yeast form to fungal form. Therefore, a low-sugar diet is necessary for the treatment of nail fungal infection.

The key to the design of the **Candida Treatment Plan** is to introduce the three key elements in various stages. If you opt to start them all at once or at the same time, it will only lead to what health influencers called a *Candida Die-Off."*

The Cleansing Phase

The *Cleansing Phase* is when you have to be on the strictest diet, consuming a lot of water to detox the body. This is to flush out your colon and quickly eliminates as many of those fungi colonies as possible.

At this stage, you must stick to a diet of raw salads and steamed veggies, along with herbs, oils, and spices to liven up your meal. This is a restrictive diet but is required only for a few days so you will end up thoroughly cleaned on the inside while feeling refreshed, light , and healthy as you move on to the next stage.

Take note that though our main concern here is the

nail fungus infection, the presence of the infection in the nail is a sign that there is an outgrowth of the fungi, which is mostly inside your digestive system.

What Food to Eat During the Cleansing Diet?

Once you have opted to start your *Antifungal Diet* with a *Cleansing Diet,* here are the foods that you must consume while on your cleansing stage.

It is preferable to use these ingredients in raw salad and steamed vegetables. You can use coconut or extra virgin oil to saute them slightly. Included in this selection of foods are herbs to make you enjoy eating while on your cleansing diet.

Vegetable

Artichoke, avocado, cucumber, raw garlic, green beans, broccoli, kale, Brussels sprouts, lettuce, okra, cabbage celery, onions, radish seaweeds, and zucchini.

- Vegetables absorbed fungal toxins and flush them out of your body.

- Eating vegetables will entirely devoid the fungi of the mold and sugar they need to exist.
- Avoid starchy root crops and all types of beans with the exception of the green beans.
- Add garlic and onion in your flavoring as they are combatants of fungi.
- "Kimchi" is probiotic and can help kill the fungi in your intestines. Raw okra and sauerkraut can work in the same way.

Herbs and Spices

Basil, cayenne, cilantro, cloves, ginger, rosemary, cinnamon oregano, black pepper ginger, cabbage celery, sea salt, black pepper, garlic, and thyme.

- Enriched with antioxidants and anti-fungal properties
- Increase blood circulation and provide relief from inflammatory symptoms
- Aids in digestion and constipation
- Most of the herbs are helpful in combating fungal infestation while

being great in livening foods when you're on a restricted diet.

Oils

Virgin Coconut Oil and Olive Oil

Coconut oil is a powerful antifungal besides being easy on the pocket.

Probiotic Foods

Another essential element involved in the treatment of the fungal infection is the consumption of Probiotics. The fungus is able to grow in your body because of the absence or lesser amount of the beneficial bacteria which are needed by your body to combat the fungi. Probiotics foods are designed to repopulate your gut with good bacteria and help you strengthen your liver.

While every person has relatively one pound of bacteria in their system, there are billions of them living in your intestine at any one time, but most of them are beneficial. By keeping your system in a healthy balance, probiotics strengthens both your immune and digestive system.

Probiotics are vital to the Candida or Fungal Treatment as it can reintroduce helpful bacteria to your gut, helping your body naturally combat the fungi. With the help of Probiotics, these useful bacteria can again rapidly grow their colony and conquer back their place in your gut. The new colony will, therefore, regulate your stomach acidity and enhance your immune system.

The Antifungal

Together with the low-sugar diet and Probiotics, another essential element to the anti-fungal treatment plan is the Antifungal. There are antifungal substances you can consume in supplement forms or add to your diet. These work effectively by breaking down the fungi cell walls, making antifungal an important part of your diet.

Popular antifungal treatments include grapefruit seed extract, garlic oil, oil of oregano, and *caprylic acid*. You can integrate antifungal to your diet however way you want. However, taking supplements is the easiest way.

The Anti-Fungus Diet

This is an important part of the diet. If you want to skip the cleansing part, then you may start here. This diet is more balanced but eliminates fruit, starchy vegetables, sugar, caffeine and any form of food with high content of glycemic. This part is designed to starve the fungus of food while providing you with the proper nutrients needed for your body.

There are few kinds of food that actually fight fungus. They are considered antifungal or Probiotics and you need to include them in your diet.

This stage can last for a few weeks to several months depending on several factors including how you follow the instruction for the diet and how effective are your Probiotics and antifungal. The severity of your fungal infection is likewise another factor to consider.

What Not to Eat

Sugar: Condiments have high sugar content and can intensify the fungus infection. Get away from sugar and also be careful of drinking diet cola as it contains *aspartame,* which can weaken your immune system.

Alcohol: Consuming too much alcohol can lead to a temporary drop in blood sugar. However, a moderate amount of it can increase it. In the long run, consuming alcohol can eventually lessen the effectiveness of insulin and can lead to a consistently high level of sugar in the blood. It likewise weakens your immunes system and increase gut permeability.

Beans: Beans are being rules out in the first stage of the diet as they are high in carb content and are hard to digest. Later, they can be reintroduced in smaller amounts. Soybeans, however, are not encouraged at all as most soy beans in north America are genetically modified.

Grains & gluten foods: People with fungus infections are highly sensitive to gluten. Foods that are by-products of corn like popcorns tend to be mold contaminated.

Fruits: The high sugar content in fruits is food for fungi to thrive on. Melon contains molds, however low sugar fruits are ok to consume during this stage.

Starchy vegetables: This group of vegetables is packed with nutrients but needs to be avoided while you still have your fungal overgrowth uncontrolled. Only once the nail fungus is fully cured can you reintroduce these gradually back into your diet.

Vinegar: Although apple cider vinegar can be helpful in fighting nail fungus, consuming large quantities can aggravate the condition. Vinegar is formed through yeast culture and can help the nail fungus grow even faster.

Caffeinated drinks: Caffeine can increase your blood pressure level and weakens the adrenals. It can also cause damage to your immune system in high quantities. Most coffee also contains molds.

Cured & processed meat: The process of cured meat will most likely contaminate the meat with molds, which increases the mold within your digestive tract when consumed. This makes it harder for you body to fight the nail fungus as it is constantly being bombarded with other molds to fight off. Processed meat should also be avoided due to the high sugar content in these meats.

Diary products: Almost all diary products need to be avoided with the exception of ghee, kefir, butter and probiotic yogurt.

Now that you know the kinds of food that you need to avoid while under treatment, you likewise ought to know the foods that you need to consume to help you fight fungi.

What To Eat

Non-starchy vegetables: By eating non-starchy foods, you are starving the invading fungi of the sugar they need to survive.

Live yogurt culture: Live yogurt brings back good bacteria to your body while holding the fungus at bay. These good bacteria helps your body keep its balance needed to fight off unwanted fungus.

Unprocessed produce: Eating fresh food prepared from scratch is the best way to ensure your food's sugar content levels as well as the possibility of mold contamination.

Herbs & Spices: A lot of herbs and spices carry antioxidants and antifungal properties. They can help inflammation as ell as improve the circulation of blood.

Oils: When possible consume cold-pressed oils and never heat oils for consumption. As heating oils destroys the nutrients as well as the anti-septic and anti-fungal properties some have.

Reintroducing Foods to Your Diet

After you have combated your fungus overgrowth through the application of low-sugar diet, Probiotics, antifungal substances and natural remedies, then this is the proper time when you can take regular food again without fearing the return of fungi invasion. However, it is vital to your health that you refrain from excess quantities of sugary junk foods again while moving on. Or else you run the risk of being prone to nail fungus infections in the future.

After getting rid of your fungal infection, it is never wise to get back to your regular diet. Remember that it's the diet that had caused the overgrowth of the fungi.

In addition, make sure that you have fully beaten the fungus and not just undergoing some temporary lapses in the symptoms. So if you are not sure of your condition, you should stick with the diet a little longer.

Foods to Reintroduce

Beans and Other Pulse

Azuki Beans, black beans lima beans, navy beans, pinto beans, carob powder, mung beans, chickpeas, and navy beans.

Vegetables

Sweet potatoes, potatoes, carrots, yams, beets, peas, winter squash, parsnips, red peppers, and yucca.

Fruits

Pears, green apples, raspberries, cranberries,

grapefruit, huckleberries, blackberries, and strawberries.

Nail fungus infection is inconvenient, agonizing and Candida Albicans is a stubborn type of fungi that is difficult to remove. However, with the popular holistic approach that is proven to be the safest, quickest, and the most effective treatment available today, you can get rid of the fungus infection in approximately 4-8 weeks through strict dietary modification and diligent application of natural anti-fungal and anti-septic remedies.

The Antifungal Application

By following the strict dietary modification, it can provide results to your physical body causing the fungus to die-off. The lack of food along with other factors is what ultimately destroys the fungus that causes the nail infection.

Take note however, that integrated within the diet regimen is the application of natural antifungals and since majority of these remedies are in food forms, they are taken as part of the diet. But in our treatment program, it is in fact the third essential element of the whole treatment program.

Soon after you start with your probiotics, which must be strictly observed for an optimal effect, try consuming two or three antifungals at the same time and get the most out of your treatment. However, you need to go slowly to avoid die-off reaction. Try rotating the use of your antifungals every 2-3 weeks, and soon as you find the right combination that works for you, stick to it. Consistently using a set of antifungals works better that continuously alternating.

How to Choose an Antifungal

There are just too many antifungals that can help you fight fungi that bring about nail fungus infection and many other forms of fungal infection. Some herbal remedies like garlic, oregano, and grapefruit seed extract are all potent antifungals.

Of the many antifungal available to us today here is the four most potent antifungal that you must not neglect.

Caprylic Acid

Caprylic acid is one of the most potent antifungal

that comes in capsule form. It is often used in the Candida Treatment. As an alternative, you can get your source of this antifungal by consuming coconut oil which contains a large amount of caprylic acid. At the start, you can take a small dose of this to avoid a Die-Off Reaction. However, as you adjust, you can take as much as 5 tablespoons per day.

Oregano Oil

You can take oregano oil either in a capsule or liquid form. If you were able to purchase it in its liquid for, the general instruction of usually 1-3 drops per day. You can take these drops diluted with water or under the tongue.

Oregano is also used against parasites and worms and therefore useful to Candida sufferers with leaky gut syndrome.

Garlic

Garlic is known to contain a compound substance named Ajoene which is another potent antifungal. A study shows that the Ajoene in garlic can destroy 09.2% of yeast including Candida.

Garlic has powerful antifungal properties which can easily destroy fungi while preserving and strengthening the good bacteria in your digestive system. This ingredient which is also easily available to us stimulates the liver and colon, detoxifying our body from a harmful substance.

Garlic is prominently used to flavor our food as it emits a strong aroma when cooked. However, uncooked, the strong smell of garlic is sure to leave a foul odor on your breath when eaten raw.

Drinking 2-4 cloves of crushed garlic combined with a minimal measure of water a day produces a great anti-fungal tonic. But then, avoid taking it on an empty stomach. Trying it with a spoonful of coconut oil will cut down the stomach burn.

To make it easier for you to take garlic, you can mince a couple o garlic cloves and drop it into a glass of water or drink with some coconut milk.

Grapefruit Extract (GSE)

Grapefruit Seed Extract is taken from the pulp and seeds of the grapefruit. GSE is known to inhibit the growth of Candida Albicans and is very popular in treatment if Candida overgrowth. Because of its potency, you need to dilute it in plenty of water and start in a small dose. If still you experience Die-Off symptoms, reduce the dose a little bit. Take note that Candida can be adaptive to GSE so you take to take this with other antifungal substances to make a set.

Other Foods That Help Fight Fungi

Coconut Oil

Coconut oil is a powerful killer of fungus and is considered one of the most potent antifungal. It contains *Caprylic acid* and *Lauric Acid*. Both help to prevent fungal overgrowth while it strengthens your immune system.

Coconut oil is a very common household ingredient ideally use in cooking, especially in frying. It is also cheap and therefore can be easily acquired in any store, grocery, or market.

Onions

Aside from the strong anti-parasitic property of

onions, it is also said to be a powerful anti-fungal remedy. It helps flush out excess fluids in the body which are useful to those who are suffering from a fungal infection as they are always experiencing water retention. Like garlic, onions can give you breathe issues. To counter the smell, eat parsley along with onions and garlic.

Seaweed

A nutrient enriched healing food, seaweeds help the body in its fight against fungi. It contains a large amount of iodine to help balance your thyroid gland. Seaweed flushes toxins and heavy metals from the body while delivering nutrients to your body.

Rutabaga

Rutabaga is one of the most powerful sources of antifungal that you can find. Although it seems to fall into the category of food to avoid like yam and potatoes, it has strong antifungal properties. If you feel it's strong for you, you can try turnips instead as it carries a milder antifungal agent. You can make a variety of food prepared from the rutabaga. You can mash it, prepare some fries out of it, or mix it in your vegetable soup.

Ginger

Ginger helps in the blood circulation and in detoxifying the liver while stimulating the immune system. It likewise helps reduce intestinal gas and has a positive effect on any inflammation caused by fungus overgrowth in the intestinal tract. Ginger tea is easy to prepare.

What you will need:

- Ginger root (1 square inch)
- Lemon extract
- Water (2 cups)

Peel the ginger off the skin and grate it. Add to the boiling water and boil for about 2 minutes. Strain and then serve hot with a slice of lemon.

Olive Oil

Olive oil contains *Oleuropein*, a substance found in both olive oil and when extracting it from oil leaf. It contains antifungal properties and helps you boosts your immune system and strengthen it to fight fungi. It is also proven to stabilize the blood sugar level which is an important factor for fungal sufferers as the high level of sugar can help feed fungal growth.

Lemon and Lime Juice

Lime and lemon juice can stimulate the peristaltic action of the colon, thereby increasing the efficient functioning of the digestive system. Both the lemons and limes are also used as great seasonings for vegetables, fish, and meat dishes.

Pumpkin Seeds

Having high content of Omega 3 fatty acids, pumpkin seeds which carries anti-fungal and antiviral properties help counter the depression symptoms brought about by fungal inflammation such as pain and skin ailments. It is also a known fact that most of us can't get enough amount of Omega 3 oils from natural sources to be able to maintain the require dietary requirement needed for thyroid health condition.

Deficiency of this nutrient can lead to lower thyroid hormone level. To boost your Omega 3 level, add pumpkin seeds to your cereals, smoothies, or salad. You can also have it as a regular snack.

Cayenne Pepper

Cayenne pepper enhances natural support to the immune and digestive system as it helps in the digestion of food. It reduces constipation by cleansing the intestines and digestive tract of fungi and toxins. Cayenne likewise increases metabolism and circulation. This somehow reduces the feeling of fatigue, one of the most common symptoms felt by a person infected with the fungus. Try using cayenne pepper liberally while preparing your meal.

Tea Tree

Tea tree, a common name for *Melaleuca* is popular for its potent antiseptic properties and capacity to heal wounds and bruises. The oil derived from this Australian native plant, *Melaleuca Alternifolia* had been widely used throughout Australia since the past century.

This plant is proven and documented to have the ability to kill many strains of fungi, bacteria, and viruses.

Doctors of functional medicine are describing

essential oils especially tea tree and oregano oil in replacement of conventional medicines as they are effective and without adverse side effects when used. It was also discovered that essential oils including these two well-known oils even carry a positive synergistic effect which means that they can help prevent antibiotic resistance from developing.

How Can Antifungal Help

Like your Probiotics, antifungals are vital in your fight against fungus. These two complements each other in the treatment. The antifungal kills the fungi while the Probiotics bring back the good bacteria which hold these fungi at bay.

There are many kinds of antifungal and all works to damage the cell walls of the fungi causing them to die. However, it's sad to say that fungus cell and human cell have similarities in the sense that both have nasty side effects. Therefore, natural antifungals are better alternatives, but for more serious infection especially in the nails, you can consult your doctor.

How to Take Antifungals?

Begin your antifungals as soon as you begin with your Antifungal Diet and start slowly in small doses. A large dose can kill too much of the fungi or yeast quickly and this could result in a severe die-off reaction. To avoid this, try to leave at least a few more days between the start of your Probiotics and your antifungal.

Additionally, it is also good to take several antifungals at the same time. There are some ideas circulating that fungi can easily adapt to a single antifungal overtime. Hence, by doing this, you can be sure that fungi will lose their adaptive ability. You can also opt to rotate every month and you don't need to fear to try a few different antifungals.

Things to Remember

To ensure that the Antifungal Treatment will work effectively for you, you have to take into consideration the following:

The Right Diet and Exercises

After the treatment, continue eating a balanced diet

rich in meat, legumes and nuts, vegetables and poultry products like chicken and eggs. Don't forget the healthy oils (organic) while avoiding carbohydrate-filled foods and sugar. This will restrict the amount of resources that can fuel the yeast and fungus present in your intestines.

In addition to the right diet, having a regular exercise will rebalance the level of neurotransmitters present in your brain. This is for the improvement of your mood.

Get Plenty of Helpful Bacteria

Continue with your probiotic (good bacteria) intake by eating cultured and fermented food. There are also available probiotic supplements in the market. These contain good bacteria that keep your gastrointestinal tract healthy and ultimately wipe out the harmful Candida Albicans.

Avoid Exposure to Chemicals

Chemicals that we used at home like perfumes, household cleaners, scents , and paints are very common in people with yeast or fungi overgrowth. Avoid contact with these chemicals to prevent the recurring presence of the fungus as much as possible.

Address Emotional and Psychological Issues

Most often, food cravings especially for sweets, are brought about by emotional dependencies. There are some techniques that can help you overcome emotional hurdles and food cravings that are unhealthy. An example is the EFT or Emotional Freedom Technique which is a psychological acupressure technique used to optimize emotional health.

Though often overlooked, emotional health is vital to physical health and healing. Without a healthy emotional state, you will find it difficult to make natural remedies work.

PREVENT NAIL FUNGUS FROM COMING BACK

A fungal infection of the nail is sometimes difficult to treat and the first attempt of medication may not work at all. A nail infection is said to be cured only when a new set of nail starts to grow again. Although it indicates that the nail is free from infection, it's always possible for the infection to return.

Possible cause for recurring nails infections are due to the following:

Repeated Exposure to Infected Surfaces
When you continually share communal spaces like the bathroom, shower room or even share personal items like shoes, socks, etc. You run the risk of nail

fungus infection to reappear as these places are highly likely to be contaminated with fungi spores.

Not Fully Treated
It could be difficult to fully treat the infection since the fungus can hide beneath the nails, making it invisible to the naked eye to detect. Though over-the-counter and natural remedies are effective, sometimes only the symptoms are relieved and they can come back soon after. It's important to be sure the fungus has been fully eliminated before treatment is stopped.

Compromised Immune System
Once your immune system is weakened due to some underlying medical condition, it could be hard to fully treat your nail infection, especially in diabetic patients when surgical treatment is not possible. Treatment must first focus on strengthening the immune system or improve the person's health condition.

Other Conditions
Conditions, which affects the flow of blood circulation like diabetes can affect your body's ability to heal after the injury brought about by the

infection. So if you have diabetes, poor blood circulation, and nerve problem, these can put you at greater risk for a repeated fungal infection.

Complications of a nail fungus infection that may arise can include the following:

- Resurgence of the fungi colony that brings about the infection
- Discoloration of the nail affected by the infection
- Permanent loss of the affected nail
- Possible spread of fungi to other parts of the body
- Paving way for bacteria to enter the body causing the development of bacterial skin infection called Cellulitis.

Nail Fungus Infection is something we just can't ignore. They are quick to spread and affect important parts of our body that leaving the infection untreated and the fungi unremoved will eventually lead to more serious medical conditions.

As this book had provided you with all the facts

necessary to know about Nail Fungus Infection, we are hoping that you will be able to easily detect the occurrence of fungi in any areas of your body especially the nails before it can affect you.

Treating this nasty disease is easier at its early stage and you can easily adapt all the possible technique you can get from here for your convenience and healing.

How to Prevent Nail Fungus Infection

Aside from proper hand and foot hygiene, prevention of nail fungus can be prevented through observance of the following health hygiene practices:

- Keep your nails short and clean at all times
- Drying your nails and spaces in between toes after taking a bath or washing your feet.
- Wear socks that are breathable
- Use antifungal powders and sprays
- Refrain from the habit of nail picking or biting
- Avoid sharing of shoes and socks

- Wash your hands often to prevent contacting infections
- Stop using nail polish and artificial nails
- See to it that you are using properly sanitized manicure and pedicure
- Avoid walking barefoot especially in public places like shower rooms.

A few lifestyle changes can help you keep nail fungus infection at bay. Additionally, keep the skin around you nails from being injured as much as possible. It is advisable to wear gloves while doing something that can expose your hands to moisture or dirt for an extended period of time, as the extended exposure allows fungi to get lodged into small spaces of the nails and skin. While gardening, use rubber gloves to keep your hands safe from fungi, as yeast and mold are commonly found in soil

CONCLUSION

Many suffer from this inconvenient fungus infection, without seeking treatment and leave their nails to gradually deteriorate over decades, but this book has shown that this does not have to be the case. If anything, the common trap of ignoring the situation will only make the condition incurable in the worse cases and in the best case require expensive medical bills and lengthy treatment terms.

In fact nail fungus is very manageable to prevent, manage and cure naturally at home. The need for professional medical help is only for those suffering the most severe cases of nail fungus infection. This book has provided you the knowledge to identify nail fungus at its initial early stages so you can take early action for quick recovery, simple actionable habits to adopt to prevent nail fungus from appearing and most importantly a completely natural method to cure your minor to moderate levels of nail fungus infection.

www.ingramcontent.com/pod-product-compliance
Lightning Source LLC
Chambersburg PA
CBHW060411190526
45169CB00002B/846